Elective Medication:

The Intricate details of Contemporary Mending

By

Dr.jerry S. Bash

Introduction

Chapter 1 :

Elective Medication and Its Set of experiences

Chapter 2 :

Elective Treatment Choices

Chapter 3 :

In general Treatment Plans and Extra Tips

Introduction

Generally, the primary reaction for Americans to a clinical issue is customary medication. There is, in any case, another choice. Elective medication is at times viewed as the most seasoned medication on the planet.

Elective medication wraps up the idea of searching out contemporary ways of managing everyday medical problems. This sort of medication looks past taking a prescription.

Individuals seeking to utilize the elective medication for two fundamental reasons. The first is a direct result of the possibility that taking meds might possibly prompt undesirable outcomes like conditions and incidental effects. The second is a direct result of the regular interest of man to track down better techniques to mend.

Elective medication envelops various treatments, like spellbinding, variety treatment, yoga, contemplation, homegrown cures, nutrient treatment, and more.

The fundamental focal point of elective medication is that life is a mix of parts that incorporates more than the treatment of illness. There is an unmistakable spotlight on carrying on with life well, joyfully, and with reason. It is accepted that this is a fundamental piece of sound living.

This guide will investigate a wide range of parts of elective medication and how it can help you. Consider utilizing the thoughts caught here next time you feel sick to start feeling improved normally.

Chapter 1
Elective Medication and Its Set of experiences

Medicines Past Ordinary

At the point when a great many people become ill, they shift focus over to regular strategies for clinical treatment for help and recuperation. There are elective strategies for treatment that are turning out to be progressively well-known.
What medicines are thought of as "ordinary?" The physician-endorsed drug, customary medical procedure, and electronic logical testing are three instances of regular medication. Most doctors support customary medication in their practices, so while seeing a specialist, it is almost certain you will be encouraged to follow ordinary clinical prompts.
The choice to utilize ordinary medication ought to be made by the patient and specialist dependent upon the situation. A modification to the kind of treatment is once in a while everything necessary to feel improved.

Elective medicines include:

. Natural cures

. Knead

. Reflection

. Needle therapy

. Some more!

Patients will frequently wind up going to elective strategies for therapy when customary techniques are incapable or a clinical issue has been

considered untreatable. Elective therapies are intended to support relief from discomfort, yet additionally, lessen pressure and strain that can demolish ongoing agony.
Elective techniques for treatment center around the entire individual; body and soul. Show strategies stringently center around the actual issues alone. For elective strategies to be powerful, the patient should be roused and put stock in the elective treatment's capacity to work.

Obviously, any serious, hazardous medical issue ought to mix traditional and elective techniques for a complete methodology. Make certain to talk with your PCP to stay away from entanglements. On the off chance that arranged well, you can make the most of the best of the two kinds of medication for a day-to-day existence that is agreeable and pleasant.

Elective Medication History and Hypothesis

Millennia prior, all medication was "elective medication." Before current science, healers would think about the full picture - profound, physical, and otherworldly - prior to recuperating a wiped-out individual.

This is one of the primary distinctions between present-day traditional medication and elective medication. Elective medication doesn't search for the moment remedy for the actual issue, rather it takes a gander at a drawn-out arrangement that incorporates the entire self.

Only years and years prior in Europe there were two sorts of healers; society healers that pre-owned old proven strategies, and expert doctors. The lower classes didn't have the cash to pay for the expert doctors, however, they utilized the people healers and it worked.

In North America, theory and religion were much of the time used to assist people healers with giving comprehensive medicines.

The customary medication that we have today has developed from the times of society healers and elective medication. Numerous customary doctors support unique

kinds of all-encompassing medicines in the general well-being plan for their patients. The explanation that elective medication has endured for the long haul is on the grounds that it works!

Antiquated Chinese Medication

Conventional Chinese medication (TCM) incorporates needle therapy, Qigong, natural

medicines, and profound back rub, and that's just the beginning. Over 25% of the total populace rehearses TCM.

A few trustworthy gatherings, for example, the World Wellbeing Association and the Public Organization of Wellbeing, view conventional Chinese medication as a reasonable option in contrast to contemporary medication.
Many pieces of TCM started above and beyond a long time back in China. The focal point of TCM is Qi (articulated "Chee"), which is the body's energy that interfaces it with our general surroundings. It is accepted that all issues and real issues are brought about by the misalignment of Qi. Needle therapy is one of the most broadly perceived techniques for bringing the Qi into an arrangement.
Natural cures are well-known in customary Chinese medication. They are utilized to unwind and quiet the patient's feelings to keep away from discouragement and give a more inspirational perspective on the disease. This helps colossally in the recuperating system. Ginseng and natural green tea are the most famous homegrown cures in China.
Workout, essentially Qigong (articulate "Chee Kung"), is additionally a significant piece of conventional Chinese medication. Qigong includes stance, reflection, and slow, determined body developments.

Tibetan Medication

Tibetan Medication is exclusively founded on homegrown cures and has been around for more than 2,500 years. It is designated "global Apparatus dad". Tibetans generally live in

India since they have been banishment since the last part of the 1950s. They practice Tibetan Buddhism.

There is a Tibetan Clinical Establishment in Northern India, where specialists reading up on Tibetan medication go for a considerable length of time prior to procuring a degree.

The basic faith in Tibetan medication is that all diseases are brought about by noxious reasoning which incorporates fear, disavowal, and need. This idea binds to the standards of the Buddhist way of thinking.

The three noxious contemplations are accepted to be brought about by terrible eating routine, unseemly way of behaving, and the irregularity of time and season. This idea is more muddled than this, however, this disentanglement will give a general feeling of it.

Fixes are join to all frameworks of the body cooperating. The disposal of sweat, defecation, and pee adds to this agreement.

Like the Chinese "Qi", the Tibetans have the Ring, which is the general life force that interfaces us with the universe.

The ring has five sorts:

1 Focused on the cerebrum. Life getting a handle on - controls breathing, keenness, sniffling, and gulping.

2 Focused on the chest. Up moving - controls verbal capacity and endurance.

3 Focused in the heart. All plaguing - controls all development like that of the openings of the body and strolling.

4 Focused on the stomach. Fire going with - controls assimilation and digestion.

5 Focused on the rectum. Descending purging - controls all that is ousted from the body, like infants, feminine blood, or semen.

Tibetan medication as a rule handles disorder conclusion by investigating the tongue and pee. The profound component is likewise affecting everything in Tibetan medication, with much consideration spent zeroing in on the kind and disposition of spirits in the body.

Native American Medication (otherwise known as Local American Medication)

North Native American clans have been rehearsing medication for what case to be more than 40,000 years. The clinical data and methods are given over from one age to another; guaranteeing the life span of the training.

A few cures are clan explicit, albeit everything ancestral medication is called Local American Medication, all things considered. Local Americans accept that man is unified with nature and that the components give strength and can fix the infection.

It is captivating to take note that while Local American medication was being drilled in North America, Conventional Chinese Medication was being polished a portion of a world away. Ayurveda (medication rehearsed in India), was likewise polished as of now and will be covered straight away.

These conventional clinical practices depend on the very essential conviction that an individual's way of life and climate ought to be thought about prior to picking a treatment way. There are unpretentious contrasts between the practices that are well-defined for the locale.

Local American medication perceives a refinement method including homegrown smoke when treatment. Medicines incorporate the utilization of sage and cedar smoke to repulse negative energy. Negative energy is viewed as the agony delivered by somebody who is sick, or the aggravation that the healer takes on themselves from their patients. Helpful touch is utilized. Singing, reciting, drums and clatters go with the recuperating during the meeting.

Ayurvedic Medication

Ayurvedic Medication is polished in India and spotlights normal recuperating. Professionals accept that the body genuinely must be adjusted, and all meds depend on vegetables and minerals, with dynamic fixings from plant alkaloids.
In Ayurvedic Medication there is the conviction that there are three components in the body, called Kapha, Pitta, and Vata, that cause sickness.

1 Kapha: This energy is brought about by the absence of settling the equilibrium in the body. These are generally called infections by Westerners.

2 Pitta: This energy upholds vision, temperature, hunger, thirst, insight, and bliss. When crooked, the results incorporate weight change, parchedness, sadness, stomach-related issues, and lack of concern.

3 Vata: This energy keeps the general harmony between the earth, sky, and world around us under control with ourselves.

Assuming that it drops out of equilibrium, the disorder is welcomed in.

Sickness is called Vyaadhi, and it is treated by zeroing in on the lopsidedness of components.

Chapter 2

Elective Treatment Choices

Homeopathy Medicines

Homeopathy is characterized as a natural arrangement of medication that depends on three principal thoughts:

1 Like fixes like

2 Insignificant dosing

3 Once cures

Elective medication generally has a minimal measure of "dynamic" fixing conceivable, with the idea of utilizing one single cure regardless of the number of side effects that are introduced. Homeopathy centers around the minimal measure of medicines for better well-being.
There are a few justifications for why homeopathy is the second most well-known type of medication (after customary medication). The most famous reasons are:

. It is very normal and safe

. The outcomes are extremely durable

. It is successful

You can take most homeopathic drugs alongside customary medication without secondary effects
It is non-habit-forming

Homeopathy is an exact science, which is the reason it at times takes more time to track down precisely the perfect medication for your sickness. Elective medication invests energy

posing inquiries about side effects and the underlying driver of the disease with an end goal to make an unmistakable determination for the issue, and treating it really.

Natural Cures

Nature gives many fixes and medicines to afflictions, everything being equal. Every locale has its own local plants that are utilized in elective medication.
While purchasing spices for restorative purposes, it is proposed that you use spices from a natural shop. Spice strength fluctuates relying upon the manner by which they are developed, so until you know all about developing strategies for restorative spices, buying from an expert is suggested.
The accompanying rundown gives natural fixes to normal sicknesses:

- Skin break out and skin weakness.

Clean up and rub a clove of garlic that has been sliced down the middle. Or on the other hand, blend lavender in with witch hazel at a 1:10 proportion. Tea tree oil can be subbed instead of lavender.

. Nervousness and stress.

Lavender unadulterated rejuvenating ointment splashed onto a cotton fabric, warmed, and collapsed into a pack. Apply to the head or neck.
Injuries and wounds.

Bubble hyssop blossoms and leaves into a color. Channel fluid, and splash a cotton pack. Apply to the wounded region by applying pressure. The hyssop, intensity, and tension mix will diminish the injury.

. Consumes.

Minor consumption can be treated with comfrey or aloe juice. Essentially rub aloe juice into the consumed region. Comfrey can be squashed into a fine powder, blended in with

equivalent pieces of dissolved beeswax, and added to vegetable oil. Stew over low intensity for 20 minutes, and afterward strain combination.

. Moles.

Either utilize a cut piece of garlic, put it straightforwardly on the mole, or, for a less rotten fix, attempt dandelion juice applied over and over the course of the day.

Natural Teas

A well-established cure, homegrown teas are utilized to calm and remember agony and stress. Numerous teas are really a color as opposed to tea. Color is a thicker tea that is spice thick and is imbued rather than soaks.

The accompanying rundown is a rundown of conditions and homegrown tea cures:

- Weakness.

Drink a color produced using bubbled stinging bramble leaves.

- Joint pain.

Drink a color of demon's hook, juniper, birch, or celery seed (not the sort on your flavor rack).

Chemotherapy incidental effects.

Drink a color of Siberian ginseng root. It alleviates the inner parts and assuages exhaustion.

- Colic in children.

Add under 10 drops of dill and fennel color to their container.

- Clogging.

Drink a liter of rhubarb root each day.

- Hack.

Drink a tea build using garlic bulbs and ribwort leaves.

- Gloom.

Drink a color day to day produced using the ground-up oat plant and St. John's mole blossoms.
Fever.

Drink a hot tea made of lemon emollient, yarrow, and ginger.

- Gas.

Drink a tea produce of caraway, fennel, ginger, and peppermint.

- Influenza side effects.

Drink a color made of Echinacea, yarrow, and catnip.

Nutrients and Minerals

Taking a nutrient enhancement isn't a replacement for eating restoratively. Nonetheless, it fills in as protection to be sure that you are getting the nutrients as a whole and minerals that your body needs.
Nutrients are crucial for the enhanced working of your body. Without adequate nutrients, for instance, your blood won't

scale. You really want nutrients to battle colds, and lift your safe framework.

It is ideal to step through a homeopathic exam to decide the nutrients that you really want. This will keep away from hazardous excess. Then, at that point, you can take the nutrients you really want exclusively, depending on the situation, and keep away from a multi-nutrient, which is crammed with fillers.

This strategy will set aside your cash, as well.

Honey bee Treatment (also known as Apitherapy)

The act of Apitherapy is the utilization of honey bee stings, honey bee dust, propolis, imperial jam, and honey to treat different ailments. While there has not been broad trying in the logical world to approve the cases of apitherapists, history demonstrates that medicines give help.

There are five lurch bee items that are utilized in apitherapy:

1 **Toxin**: A professional will help the patient in permeate or being stung by honey bees in the impacted region. The toxin is utilized to give help to conditions like tendonitis, Numerous Sclerosis, and degenerative bone
2 **sickness**. It works in light of the fact that the toxin is a characteristic calming which is more strong than others accessible to customary medication like hydrocortisone. You

should get tried to be sure that you are not sensitive to beestings preceding presenting yourself to honey bee toxin.

3 **Dust**: A characteristic energy supplement that is likewise utilized as a sensitivity to pollen help. Dialing back the improvement of wrinkles is likewise accepted.

4 **Crude Honey**: A wellspring of speedy energy, crude honey is utilized for some fixes. It might in fact be utilized as an ointment on top of a fresh injury to keep away from the spread of microscopic organisms.

5 **Illustrious Jam:** This is the smooth white substance that the working drones produce to take care of the sovereign. While unverified, this substance is utilized as a wonderful help and is accepted to assist with bringing down cholesterol.

6 **Propolis**: This is the paste used to hold the hives together and make fixes. Propolis is produced using the sap of poplar and conifer trees. It is utilized to make lip emollients and treatments and is viewed as a cell reinforcement.

Iridology

Iridology is the name for the act of deciding an individual's harmfulness in view of the shade of their iris. This idea returns to Sweden and Hungary where doctors utilized it to measure sickness in their patients.

For quite a long time, renowned doctors and researchers, as far as possible back to the Greek doctor Hippocrates, have found individuals with wounds get dark imprints across the iris of their eye. These imprints later vanish as the individual's infirmities recuperate.

In this day and age, iridology is utilized as a deterrent measure to check in the event that there is an adjustment in an individual's well-being. Tragically iridology can't be utilized to acknowledge a particular sickness.

The manner by which iridology is polished today is that the shaded piece of the eye (the iris) is painstakingly shot utilizing major areas of strength for a focal point. It is effortless, and it requires about an hour to finish. The photographs are then extended, and a prepared proficient iridologist reads up it for indications of conceivable sickness.

Indeed, even customary specialists utilize the eyes as an early advance notice indication of terrible things happening within the body. This study is only the more engaged investigation of the iris while searching for indications of degenerative medical problems.

Contemplation in Recuperating

Contemplation is an expertise that is mastered. When you know how to do it appropriately, it tends to be utilized to work on your personal satisfaction and well-being incredibly.
The advantages of contemplation are an expanded degree of energy, a more uplifting outlook, superior invulnerable well-being, better rest quality, and the easing back of the maturing system.
To exploit the greatest advantage, contemplate for no less than 20 minutes out of every day preceding sleep time.

Follow these means for contemplating. In the first place, plunk down and settle in a calm room. Keep your back and neck straight, and clear your psyche with the goal that you are zeroing in on the current second.
Then, at that point, become mindful of your relaxation. Take all through your mouth, and focus on your stomach rising and falling.
On the off chance that considerations come into your head, recognize them and let the cross your thoughts. Stay aware of your breathing and unwind. Assuming your considerations divert you, don't get baffled. Just get once again to zero in on your relaxing.
At the point when your time contemplating is done, become mindful of your environmental elements and stand up leisurely.
Contemplation is a superb approach to immediately loosen up yourself and return to your being. It is the ideal enhancement to any treatment, both other options and contemporary.

This profound unwinding procedure will assist with eliminating pressure and tension from life. Diminished pressure can help with recuperating.

Jujitsu and Yoga

Judo is an exceptionally delicate type of activity that anybody can do. Since a great many people invest a large portion of their energy sitting, customary activity really must turn into a piece of their everyday daily schedule. Yoga can turn into that day-to-day development.

Practice assists by working on circulatory capability, diminishing migraine strain, bringing down blood with pressuring, and wiping out constant back and neck torment.

Judo is a progression of developments and stretches that anybody can do from any position, in any event, sitting. The activity will further develop stance, endurance, and adaptability.

Developments in Yoga are slow and think, and simple to learn. Going to a class is the most effective way to learn Judo. Try not to stress over not being in shape; Judo is known to be an activity that is finished by a wide range of individuals, all things considered.

Yoga

Yoga is an extraordinary activity movement for a wide range of individuals. It is easy, however, you in all actuality do need to find out about it. The primary objective of yoga is to make a reasonable connection between your physical and psychological wellness.

Yoga is a lifestyle that is conveyed over the course of the day, not only while in yoga class. Yoga makes you attention to yourself and your everyday life. This is an intense change for many individuals who frequently live progressing automatically.

You can conclude how you need to utilize yoga, for its essential motivation behind uniting brain and body, or to a greater extent an exhausting movement for practice purposes.

In yoga, it is ideal to begin at the most reduced level conceivable and move gradually up as you foster strength and understanding. Very much like most different things, it is critical to know the primary ideas prior to stretching out into a more troublesome area,

You can take educator-drove classes, or advance at home through the wide assortment of DVDs.

Bikram Yoga

Bikram yoga is otherwise called "hot yoga", basically on the grounds that rehearsed in space has been warmed to the north of 115 degrees. Hot yoga basically centers around stretches and balance. It additionally is loaded up with moves that make tension in the body that blocks the flow. By going through the developments, the steady development of strain made by extending is then delivered, giving a surge of blood through the veins. This is accepted to wipe them out.

There are 26 postures in hot yoga. The reason for the hot climate in Bikram yoga is the glow warms the body's muscles and ligaments which helps with adaptability.

There are a couple of tips for individuals thinking about this kind of yoga. To begin with, on the grounds that it is drilled in a hot room, you will perspire a ton. Wearing suitable light clothing is ideal. It is likewise really smart to drink a lot of water preceding your meeting.

Hatha Yoga

The fundamental focal point of Hatha yoga is breathing, contemplation, and stance. The act of this type of yoga is ideal for individuals that are different from it. Hatha yoga has to a greater extent a solid accentuation on the psychological part of reflection, blended in with yoga.

Karma Yoga

The Karma type of yoga arranges the profound and actual universes. The basics of Karma yoga are situated in the Hindu way of thinking and religion. It consolidates two contending ways of thinking on the planet; from the West - that life ought to be joy based, and from the East - that life ought to be lived for information. The two speculations are mixed in karma.
Your power development is dependent on how you carry on with your life. Terrible karma comes from carrying on with your life with the end goal of cash, riches, and material

belongings. Great karma comes from carrying on with your life for bliss and love.
Karma yoga assists you with zeroing in on your life as you find out about your life objectives and helps guide you in the correct heading.

Neuro Semantic Programming (NLP)

Neuro Phonetic Programming can be viewed as the force of positive ideas and petitions. It is legitimate all through science and medication that had an inspirational perspective, viewpoint, and a positive emotionally supportive network encompassing you is one of the best elective prescriptions that anyone could hope to find.

NLP is a strategy for programming your contemplations to be positive. This procedure centers around your sub-cognizant and your fantasies. It is basic to really accept that you can recuperate yourself for NLP to work.
How would you rehearse NLP? To start with, take a procedure that you know makes progress in different parts of your life, and apply it to your recuperating cycle. You totally should have confidence in your body's mending skill for everything to fall into place.

Solid and Skeletal Elective Medication

There are various other elective medicines for the skeletal and strong frameworks of the body. They include:

1 Kinesiology

Experts test the different muscles all through the body to decide regions that are not adjusted as expected, and afterward reestablish harmony by utilizing various methods.

2 Message

Message is the utilization of strain to knead the connective tissue inside the body. This considers the body to be more adaptable and be adjusted appropriately. Rolfing will give more energy and less tension.

3 Knead Treatment

Knead treatment is utilized to separate the raise muscles, and to retrain the muscles. It works the tendons, ligaments, and delicate tissue muscles. Knead treatment increments dissemination and works on relaxing.

4 Variety treatment

Variety treatment utilizes variety and light to treat afflictions. Frequently viewed as a corresponding treatment, a variety of treatments is utilized notwithstanding other treatments. There are seven varieties that relate to the frequency habitats of the body. Each tone is coordinated with a locale of the body.

5 Attractive energy

The utilization of attractive energy fields too, as attractive advisors accept, to control cells with attractive energy. They likewise accept they can re-energize cells. Attractive energy can likewise increment blood stream that will then decrease scars on organs, give headache help, and another repeating torment.

6 Craniosacral treatment (CST)

The craniosacral framework is the films and liquid that envelopes the cerebrum and spinal line. By applying delicate strain to the head, the cadence of the craniosacral framework can be assessed and somehow or another controlled. This works on the stream and capability of the focal sensory system. This treatment is utilized in elective medication as a protection measure. Proficient craniosacral treatment specialists accept they can find and deliver energy pimples by unblocking them and realigning the neck.

Needle therapy

In needle therapy, flimsy needles are embedded into the skin to draw nerve excitement at pinpointed areas around the body. Needle therapy is a Chinese operation that includes Dao - the backer for living in equilibrium and control, with yin and yang - two life components that are pairing powers that when adjusted give great well-being and joy. Needle therapy brings helps agony, helps respiratory diseases and eases migraines and ulcers, among other actual issues. It additionally balances the qi life force.

Reiki

Reiki is the act of moving mending energy from the healer's hands to the evil individual. This should be possibly involved and in good ways. The healer is accepted to be loaded with general energy. It is imagined that the specialist can utilize Reiki energy to adjust the recurrence of the air. Recuperating is accomplished first truly, then, at that point, inwardly, and lastly profoundly.

Gems: An Instrument for Mending

Gems have for some time been related to elective recuperating. A precious stone is made when glasslike is shaped by minerals being organized in an exact example.
Quartz is the most well-known precious stone. The conviction behind the utilization of gems is that hindered energy will be delivered when the precious stone is put at explicit focus around the body.

Chapter 3

In general Treatment Plans and Extra Tips

Five Methods for bringing the Brain, Body, and Soul Together

Brain and body are effectively characterized, however, what is the "soul" of you? The soul, or soul, can be viewed as the piece of you that is in a deep sense energetic. What makes you enthusiastic? The following are a couple of thoughts that can assist you with choosing:

1 Anticipate something that you can expect.

2 Make a blissful spot where you can go when you contemplate.

3 Think back to your victories.

4 Find something that eases your pressure and do it.

5 Investigate your future objectives - not cash related.

Kama-Sutra

The Kama-Sutra is an old text about sexual well-being that was composed at some point between the first and sixth 100 years in India. There are 35 parts that cover everything from how to track down a spouse, to how to act in bed, to how to make yourself appealing to other people.

Areas of the book cover the connection between diet and sexual prosperity. Healthy, nutritious food varieties are explicitly referred to. Receptors are suggested, through food, for expanded sexual joy.

Breathing procedures are anxious. This helps ease pressure and works on by and large sexual well-being.

Feng Shui

Feng Shui is the idea of being natural and regular examples and environmental elements in our homes and day-to-day existences. This will carry congruity and quiet arrangement with the world.

Feng Shui unites the entirety of the components. Fire, earth, air, water, and the extra "metal", are addressed inside the

home by the choice of lighting, fragrances, sounds, and the situation of furniture and apparatuses.

The fundamental idea is that the qi, or life force, should have the option to move uninhibitedly in a room. Accordingly, the area of furniture, for instance, is significant.

Chiropractics

Chiropractics is an option restorative practice that is currently thought to be regular. The principal hypothesis behind

chiropractics is that the vertebrate of the spine isn't in the arrangement. It is accepted that this misalignment causes numerous sicknesses and problems all through the body.
Bone and joint specialists use strain to realign and change the spine. Most bone and joint specialists likewise take a gander at the entire picture - stress, way of life decisions, and by and large well-being - while suggesting treatment.
Bone and joint specialists have been known to recuperate many clinical issues
through their work on understanding's backs. Asthma, headaches, joint inflammation, and more issues can be generally emphatically affected.
This treatment is protected and generally reasonable. It is non-hesitant. Going to a bone and joint specialist will surely require ordinary visits on the grounds that your issues won't be completely treated in only one meeting.

Biofeedback

Biofeedback is a device used to check interior capability, then, at that point, decide treatment, and afterward measure on the off chance that treatment is working appropriately. Like a thermometer or scale to gauge the body weight or on the other hand in the event that there is a fever, biofeedback is gathered through devices.
The body capability that it is estimating is an action that one can't intentionally control, for example, pulse and mind frequencies.

The primary suggestion in elective well-being for biofeedback is normally unwinding. This decreases the pulse, quiets the mind, and significantly influences the impacted pieces of the body.

Involving Elective Medication in Kids

Now and again customary medicines are impossible for kids. One illustration of when elective prescriptions are a practical choice for kids is the point at which they will not take their non-prescription drug. They may be more able to take a natural cure since it is something else.
Consider talking about with your ordinary specialist these beneficial medicines for kids:

. Needle therapy

The needles discharge endorphins to the mind which can assist jokes with asthma, and lessen different agonies.

. Entrancing

This procedure could give a youngster more discipline with respect to the standard organization of their regular medicine.

. Unwinding methods and back rub

This can assist messes around with asthma and manage choking aviation routes. Back rub can assist with loosening up the pressure encompassing asthma too. Breathing procedures can assist jokes around with feeling in charge of their relaxation. Jokes with additional serious sicknesses, for example, diabetes and disease can utilize the loosening up advantages of back rub to ease pressure and assist with keeping an inspirational perspective.

Continuously do a lot of examinations and talk with your youngster's primary care physician prior to starting any elective clinical procedures.

Orientation Explicit Elective Medication

People each have their own clinical requirements intended for their orientation. It is astute to consider what areas of elective medication are best designed for your orientation.

For ladies, issues connected with the feminine cycle -, for example, customary period and PMS are generally hotly debated issues. For these issues, ladies have the accompanying homeopathic choices:

. Needle therapy

. Chinese restorative spices and natural teas

. Osteopathy

. Gem treatment

. Yoga

. Entrancing

For men, issues around prostate well-being and by and large prosperity can include an elective methodology. Men have these options:

. Yoga

. Needle therapy

. Natural medicines

All types of people need to really focus on their well-being. A proactive, homeopathic methodology will guarantee a blissful, solid life.

Homeopathic Weight reduction

There are elective procedures that can be utilized in the battle to lose undesirable pounds. Obviously, very much like in ordinary medication, there is no enchanted pill.

Nonetheless, the norm "eat well, be the more dynamic" procedure of getting in shape can be improved with elective medication.
To start with, you can think about yoga. This exercise is slow and determined, yet the outcomes can be emotional. At the point when rehearses sincerely and consistently, you can acquire muscle and lose fat.

Needle therapy can diminish food desires that are subverting your weight reduction endeavors. Teas can assist with checking desires as well as detoxifying the body.
Follow these tips to get thinner with elective medication:

1 Utilize a juicer to drink your leafy foods.

2 Add Omega-3 to your refreshments.

3 Visit a homeopathic specialist for a nourishing assessment.

4 Contact a botanist for suggestions on elective teas.

5 Think about taking ox-like or shark ligament.

6 Entrancing can be utilized for social alteration.

Elective Medication and Malignant growth

Individuals with malignant growth frequently search for feasible choices that they can use to battle this illness. hadly, there is no remedy for the disease. Traditional therapies are the most forceful, and keeping in mind that other options and customary medication ought to cooperate to give an exhaustive clinical encounter, as of now they don't.

You can utilize elective medication to enhance your traditional disease medicines. Here are probably the best corresponding elective medicines:
Needle therapy: Assists with sickness, sleepiness, torment, and migraines.

Natural cures: Ginger, for one's purposes, is useful in managing queasiness and spewing brought about by chemotherapy.
Hyperbaric oxygen treatment is at present being concentrated as an integral therapy for radiation treatment.
Rub eases weakness.

One of the greatest advantages of free therapies is that the debilitated individual can assume command of their circumstance and treatment, regardless of whether simply in a little manner. This helps the patient's opportunities for endurance and works on personal satisfaction.
Likewise, with any clinical treatment, talk with your PCP before self-treating. Hazardous and counterproductive aftereffects can result on the off chance that treatment isn't strongly arranged.

What Occurs in an Elective Treatment Meeting?

It, most importantly, is vital to pick the right expert for you. While choosing your ideal expert, make certain to audit their qualifications since there are numerous deceitful specialists in the elective clinical world.
Follow these tips to track down the ideal specialist:

1 Search the telephone directory and online for neighborhood experts. Select a neighborhood gathering of professionals.
2 Research this gathering of professionals to figure out their experience, training, style, and whatever else you can about them.
3 Figure out what associations they are partnered with. The more exchange gatherings, the better.
4 Teach them to ask what explicit experience they have with your sort of circumstance.
5 Ask what the treatment interaction is for your given circumstance.

The focal point of an elective medication meeting is different than what happens in a conventional clinical meeting. Here, the professional will need to find out about you in general individual, in addition to the particular area of injury or concern.

Instructions to Turn into an Elective Clinical Expert

Could it be said that you are pondering turning into an elective clinical professional? The calling is fulfilling and fascinating and furnishes you with the chance to help individuals. By giving an elective medication administration, you will have an effect on the planet.

To begin with, you should figure out which kind of elective medication you need to rehearse. Elective medication is separated into seven classifications:

1 Dioelectricmagnetic applications

2 Diet

3 Sustenance

4 Way of life changes

5 Home grown medication

6 Manual recuperating

7 Natural medicines

To turn into an expert elective medication professional, you should effectively finish a licensed program at an enlisted school. There are many schools that have some expertise in some space of elective medication.
Tutoring is serious, and a decent program will incorporate long periods of study and practice, as well as temporary position insight.

Whenever you have finished school and practicum work you will actually want to rehearse your field of concentration all alone.

Paying for Elective Medication

Costs for elective medicines differ. Most medicines are not covered by protection, so examining genuine costs before delivering administrations from a practitioner is significant.
The most vital phase in figuring out how to pay for treatment is to call your insurance agency to check whether they will cover your treatment meeting. Assuming they do cover, figure out the particulars. What number of meetings? Is there a particular sort of treatment that is just covered?
At the point when you meet your professional, perhaps the earliest inquiry to pose is in the event that they acknowledge your kind of protection. On the off chance that you are not utilizing protection, you should resolve an elective installment.

Conclusion

In North America, elective medication has encountered an expansion in prominence lately. Obviously, there is discussion encompassing the two major kinds of medication; customary and conventional.

With each of the superb advantages of elective medication, there are a few dangers related to it. The following dangers ought to be considered prior to utilizing elective medication:

1 Hazardous, insufficient, untested substances

2 Paying attention to misrepresented cases of security by a few deceitful organizations

3 Renouncing traditional medicines for

difficult ailments to utilize an elective treatment.

4 Not revealing the synchronous utilization of both traditional and elective medicines, perhaps making a negative well-being circumstance

Perceiving potential dangers in elective medicine is significant. Similarly as with anything, in the event that a treatment, item, or substance sound like it is unrealistic - then, at that point, it presumably is!

Continuously research the treatment or substance, as well as any specialists that you are contemplating utilizing. Actually take a look at certifications and references, if conceivable. Since a large part of the elective medication world is unregulated, there are cheats out there that you should be tired of.

Assuming you are cautious about what you put in your body, and the sorts of outside treatment you request, you can go with taught decisions that will help your well-being extraordinarily.

The best methodology is a decisively arranged approach that you make and examine with your PCP. In the event that you are not happy talking with your customary clinical specialist about enhancing with elective medication medicines, then, at

that point, find one that is open mined about this kind of treatment. You will be cheerful if you did.

Just once you have researched every one of the different elective medicines from around the world will you have a full comprehension of what choices are out there. The web is a great spot to start your examination process.

www.ingramcontent.com/pod-product-compliance
Lightning Source LLC
LaVergne TN
LVHW052107160826
845678LV00015B/3419

* 9 7 9 8 3 6 1 1 8 2 3 3 6 *